PRAYING PRACTITIONER

Testimonies and Teachings

Dr John W Holladay

DEDICATION

This book is dedicated to you, the medical practitioner or caregiver, who desires to give more than medicine to your patient. This book was birthed out of numerous and spontaneous encounters of praying for patients that co-workers and I experienced while working in our downtown pharmacy.

This book is dedicated to you, the medical practitioner or caregiver, to encourage you to step out of your comfort zone and pray for your patients. The most difficult patient to pray for is the first one. Whether you are in a large teaching hospital in New York City or a small dental practice in Rural Town, USA, Father God is there (see Jeremiah 23:23-24) and is eagerly awaiting your participation.

This book is dedicated to my Spirit-filled co-workers who "lays hands on the sick" and see them recover: Susan, who is my amazing wife, Laney, Teresa, Ann, and numerous pharmacy students have all prayed for patients and seen the Father heal. Dr. Mag, Linda and Liz are friends who never miss a chance to pray for those in need of the Father's touch. Thank you all for your mentorship.

I wish to thank my earthly, Spiritual fathers, who have all in some way contributed to the experiences described in this book: Edward, who is my Dad, Pastor H. Sorrells, Dr WC Smith, Pastor Sims, Pastor Coker and both Pastors Kgosana, Dr Peter Wyns, Pastor Jock, Pastor Todd, Mr Lyles – the best Sunday School teacher ever, Hap and Sue, El Patron Tindall, Jess and Ole Doug.

I give all the honor and glory and praise to our Father, who is in Heaven and dwells in unapproachable light. Thank you, Father for giving me the opportunity to assist in Your work. Blessed be the name of the Lord.

I wish to thank my parents, Edward and Betty, for rearing my sister, Steph, and me in a Christian home. Thanks, Mom, for choosing life! And thank you, Mr Bobby, for your stand for Christ.

Many blessings to you, my medical colleagues. Please give your patients more than medicine.

Contents

Preface

"I urge you, brothers and sisters,
by our Lord Jesus Christ and by the
love of the Spirit, to join me in my
struggle by praying to God for me."

Romans 15:30

While practicing pharmacy for more than 30 years, there have been innumerable times when patients and caregivers have mentioned to me at the end of a conversation to, "keep us in your prayers." No matter the walk of life, it is very likely that some variance of this request has been spoken to all of us. Usually, this is an expression of concern and vulnerability from those who need a touch from the Lord. In the Southeast USA, where my wife and I live, this phrase is usually answered with, "We sure will."

But do we? And how exactly do we keep someone in my prayers? What type of prayer do we need to pray to satisfy my hasty agreement to keep someone in my prayers? And how long do we need to pray to qualify for having kept someone in my prayers?

The motivations of asking for prayer are as varied as the desired outcomes. Sometimes, patients simply want to know that someone cares about them and is in their corner. This type of scenario is one in which the problem does not need to be fixed but rather esoterically understood. Other times, patients know that an impending procedure, surgery, or diagnostic is about to occur, and they want a comprehensive and flawless process. Then, there are times when patients realize that if a clear touch from God Almighty does not occur, they are facing the unimaginable.

The goal of this book is to educate, encourage, exhort, and commission the healthcare practitioner to begin praying for their patients (Rom 1:11). Each chapter has a sentinel scripture to consider while the reader spends time in that chapter. Some of the chapters are actual testimonies from experiences at my site of pharmacy practice, and other chapters contain teachings and areas of interest regarding praying for patients. Each chapter concludes with 2 questions to think through, or hopefully, to be discussed in an intra-office intensive study on that particular topic. Five suggested scriptures for further study and contemplation are also provided.

I encourage you to question and think about the issues and explanations in this book. With this mindset, thoroughly consider each chapter and determine its relevance to your healthcare practice. Only those sentences or phrases referenced as quotes from Bible translations are Scripture. All else is human opinion and interpretation.

Several scriptures give us insight into "keeping us in your prayers". Romans 1:9-10, 1 Thessalonians 1:2, and Acts 12:12, are among the examples. When we keep someone in our prayers, we are not necessarily repeating the same phrase, "Lord, please heal Mrs. Jones", hundreds of times a day for weeks. I believe we should have a time of intentional intercession for Mrs. Jones in which we describe to Father God our compassion for her, our desire to see her completely healed, and our desire to see Father God receive all the glory.

Once we have thoroughly laid out our heart before God about Mrs. Jones, we should transition to thanking God for hearing our prayer and for the upcoming answer to our prayer. All the while, we realize and accept that God will likely answer in a way we do not expect. We pray, He answers.

This book is written primarily for Christian healthcare workers; and more broadly, for those healthcare workers who believe in the Almighty God in Heaven, the God of Abraham, Isaac, and Jacob. If you are a healthcare practitioner who does not believe in God, I encourage you to read this book with a skeptical eye. Do not take my word as fact. Test it out yourself. Either Father God is who He claims to be in His Holy Scriptures and can do what He said, or He is simply one of many gods available today in our postmodern culture.

I believe the God of the Holy Bible is who He says He is. I have seen too much and experienced too much to deny Him and what He is able to do. He is our Creator. He is our Father. He is our Shepherd. He is our Healer. He is our Redeemer.

Father God also wants us to be involved with His ministry. The prophet Isaiah responded to the question from God, "Whom shall I send? And who will go for Us?" (Is. 6:8) I do not believe at all that Abba Father was clueless about whom to send. God knows all and sees all. (Jn. 16:30). I believe God was smiling at Isaiah as He asked His question. This reminds me of a football coach who has given a rousing pregame speech and then asks his players, "Who's ready to play?!"

The Lord is asking all of us in the healthcare fields, "Whom shall I send?" As disciples of Jesus, among other directives, we are commanded to heal the sick. (Matt. 10:8). Healing the sick has a special place for us in healthcare and is the primary reason that we entered healthcare. People are hurting. People are confused and anxious about their disease. People are losing hope. The Father is asking healthcare workers, "Who will go for Us?" Let us resolve to pray for those whom the Father sends our way.

My prayer for you is that this book will help you and your office move into a place of prayer for your patients and be guided by the Spirit of the Lord in this endeavor. Many blessings to you as you serve Father God in healthcare as a Praying Practitioner.

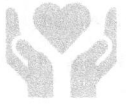

CHAPTER 1

Testimony of Immediate Healing

"When Jesus landed and saw
a large crowd,
He had compassion on them
and healed their sick."

Matthew 14:14

On one occasion at the pharmacy, a husband and wife came in to get their annual influenza vaccines. After the appropriate paperwork and billing were completed, we all moved over to the immunization area. I am usually a free-talker and started with my usual jokes to lighten the mood. Who enjoys getting jabbed with a needle anyhow? A little humor tends to help ease the anxiety of the needle stick.

"Hey, I have good news!" Usually, the patient will respond with the baited question, "What is it?"

"I have never missed, so there is nothing to worry about!" At this flat joke, the husband giggled nervously and looked at his wife who sat motionless.

I decided to inject the husband first. Men, in general, squirm a little more than women during the injection process, but his receptiveness to my simple joke led me to believe I should start with him. After plopping the empty syringe in the sharps container, he commented on my excellent technique, clearly intending to disarm his wife.

Her sleeve was already rolled up and she had not budged. I asked her to relax her arm which she held as a Marine would at platoon attention. Anyway, I had other things waiting on me, so I injected the vaccine, took off my gloves and described the necessary wait required post-injection. She grabbed her purse and swiftly left the husband in the dust.

The couple merged into the small crowd at our soda fountain restaurant while I went back to the waiting prescriptions. Then, the Divine Appointment happened.

The wife came back to the consult window of the pharmacy and asked to speak to me. Usually, this is not a good sign as it is often indicative of a complaint. "Yes ma'am, do you have a question about the injection?" I asked with a broad smile that I hoped did not betray my true feelings. She responded, "No, I want to talk to you about this rash on my arm." I noticed thousands of perfectly formed goose bumps all over her otherwise flawless skin. My medical training engaged in my mind to offer the standard questions. How long have you had these? When did they start? Do you believe these appeared after the injection? Do they itch? What remedies have you tried, whether over-the-counter or prescription?

Praying for this lady did not cross my mind immediately. I spent most of that time praying for me. Honestly, she was a bit intimidating with those piercing eyes. However, Holy Spirit told me to "probe further." My first question was, "When did this start?" At this point, the woman of steel began to melt. Tears formed in her eyes. Generally, this is a spot-on indication that I have hit the target with the correct question and the Spirit is working on that target. "About 2 months ago."

Of course, I wanted to know what happened 2 months ago, and so I asked. She replied, "My sister died of COVID-19." OK, Lord, what do I do next? Learning to develop "dual listening" is critical to effectively praying for your patients. Listen to the patient and listen to Holy Spirit as He directs, corrects, and adds details. I sensed "grief" was the culprit.

"Can I pray for you?" flew out of my mouth before I could internally debate the question. "Yes, please. My husband said you would. And God told me to come over here and talk to you. But I was hesitant… " My first interpretation of the look in her eyes was that she was previously hurt or offended by someone who looked like me and talked like me.

I would like to pause this true story to state a few words on this subject. Many of our patients have been taken advantage of or treated as ignorant by previous encounters with those in authority or in a position of knowledge. My fellow healthcare workers, please humble yourselves and do not take up offense from those who may look at you with hesitation or distrust. Stay the course and stick with plan. In the end, the patient will know, and not just guess, who you are by your actions and fruit you produce. The result of this course of action will be an appreciative and loyal patient. "A good name is more desirable than great riches; to be esteemed is better than silver or gold." (Prov. 22:1).

I asked the patient in this story if I could lay my hands on her forearm and she agreed. Jesus is our trailblazer here. One characteristic continually preceded His healings of all kinds: Compassion. "When Jesus landed and saw a large crowd, He had compassion on them and healed their sick." (Matt. 14:14) The first step is to start with compassion. Realize that the person wants to be heard and understood. They seek empathy. They seek compassion. I began the prayer by pronouncing a blessing over the patient. She is God's daughter. She is the apple of His eye. Father God takes delight in her.

Then I asked the patient if she would allow Jesus to come into the memory of her sister's death and bring healing to that area. She nodded in the affirmative and reached for more tissues. In this type of prayer, I am not commanding or demanding anything. I am simply ushering the patient into the presence of the Word of God, the Christ of the Lord, Jesus of Nazareth. Jesus is the Healer, as the scripture at the beginning of this chapter testifies. She stood there crying while a smile began to develop. She said she felt the love of the Lord and His warmth soothing her body. Healing from grief was occurring.

After saying amen, and providing more tissues, we watched the bumps disappear. She gave her grief to Jesus, and in its place, Jesus gave her peace. She let the grief go and chose the peace and love of Jesus instead. Her husband slipped up behind her and touched her side. She spun around and fell into his arms, still crying. He glanced at me with a thankful nod and slowly walked her out of the store.

What were the ingredients of this Divine Appointment? I was willing and available. I listened to the Holy Spirit and followed His guidance. I recognized there is no recipe or formula. Each opportunity requires a unique approach. Of course, there are similarities with many healing prayers, but each instance will be distinct. "The wind blows where it wishes, and you hear the sound of it, but cannot tell where it comes from and where it goes…"(Jn. 3:8 NKJV). Whatever else happened that day was forgotten by the time I reached home. It was all I wanted to share with my wife. I pray that you all experience the joy of relating the results of a Divine Appointment that only Father God could have arranged.

"What do you think?"

Matthew 21:28

1. Describe to your group a time when you were compelled to pray for one of your patients. What was the outcome?

2. What are some lessons of the encounter described in this chapter that will help you to pray for your patients in your practice?

Go Deeper

John 5:5-9
Matthew 15:30-31
John 14:12-15
Matthew 10:8
Acts 3:6-8

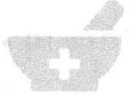

CHAPTER 2

Scriptural Basis for Healing

"If you love Me,
keep My commands."

John 14:15

No matter the denomination, all Christians should agree on several sentinel scripture passages. One of them is the response of Jesus to His disciples when they asked Jesus to teach them how to pray in Luke Chapter 11. Jesus said in verse 2, "When you pray, say: 'Our Father in heaven, Hallowed be Your name. Your kingdom come. Your will be done, On earth as it is in heaven.'" (NKJV)

Our Father in Heaven

Immediately introduced in this scripture is the concept of God as our Father. There may be many people who do not have fond memories of their earthly father. Some even have no memory of their father. A deeper dive into the nature of our Heavenly Father can be found in Luke 15, in the parable of the lost son, or as The Passion Translation titles it, "The Loving Father." In this parable, the father pursues both the wayward, rebellious son and the obedient, but distant, older son. He loves them equally and wants His best for them. Father God wants the very same for you and the person for whom you are praying.

Hallowed Be Your Name

Next, we see Jesus giving glory to the Father. Psalm 103:19 declares, "The Lord has established His throne in heaven, and His kingdom rules over all." From the original Hebrew, "all" is translated into English as "all." So what is left out of "all"? All is everything and excludes nothing.

God has the final say. This firm foundation is repeated in 1 Chronicles 29:12, "Wealth and honor come from you; you are the ruler of all things. In your hands are strength and power to exalt and give strength to all." It withstands the scrutiny of logic that physical healing is included somewhere in the vastness of "all."

Your Kingdom Come, Your Will Be Done, On Earth as It Is in Heaven

What is going on in God's kingdom? Dallas Willard mentions in his book, The Divine Conspiracy, that the "Kingdom of God is the range of God's effective will. It is where what God wants done is done." This leads us to the question, "What is His will?" While the answer to this question is too immense to fathom, let us focus on the issue of sickness and disease.

Isaiah 25:8 states "He will swallow up death forever. The Sovereign Lord will wipe away the tears from all faces; He will remove His people's disgrace from all the earth." Revelation 21:4 echoes this verse. "There will be no more death or mourning or crying or pain, for the old order of things has passed away."

Disease and sickness are at least one cause of the signs listed above. Let us consider pain. There will be no pain in the presence of the Lord when the time comes in which His dwelling place is with us. In the presence of the Lord, there is no crying. There is no sorrow. Rather, there is love, joy, and peace. Thus, when we pray for the Lord's kingdom to come (to reign) on earth, we should realize that healing comes with this plea.

In God's original design, disease was non-existent. God did not allow sin into the world. Humans did. We listened to the father of lies and looked away from God to our own wants and desires (see Genesis Chapter 3). This allowed sin to enter the world. One of the mechanisms used by the enemy of our God to destroy the creation made in the image of God was to inflict that creation with disease. Then, God allowed humans to experience the consequence of the blasphemous decision to believe the lie instead of the truth of God.

A publication from the Department of Theology at the University of Notre Dame (Journal for the Study of Pseudepigrapha. 28.1. 2018. p.

1-23) enlightens us on the potential origin and treatment of disease dating back to the time of the Biblical Noah. Ancient Jewish writings portray Noah as receiving advice from the angels of God regarding natural remedies to combat diseases that were inflicted on Noah's subsequent generations by evil spirits.

Contemporary charismatic churches have been awarded the reputation of believing evil spirits are behind most of the maladies in our world today. Yet, in the Book of Jubilees, Jewish scholars who are far distant from the theology of the contemporary charismatic church, attribute disease to the works of evil. Diseases today are propagated in many ways, but the root of every disease may be traced back to the decision to disobey God.

In the presence of God Almighty, disease and illness cannot exist. Our God dwells in unapproachable light. (1 Tim. 6:16) There is no darkness or shadow of turning in our God. (Jas. 1:17). The Word (Jesus Christ) is the same yesterday, today and forever. (Heb. 13:8) Thus, there is no time in which God will tolerate disease and sickness in His Kingdom. Since we have rebelled from God's Kingdom and decided to establish our own kingdom (again, Genesis chapter 3), He will allow diseases and sicknesses into our kingdom because of our ancestors' decision. And He allows us to freely seek remedies to these illnesses that we experience in our kingdom.

These remedies include physical therapy, exercise, proper nutrition, and medications. It is time we institute prayer as the first remedy applied to disease. God is able to wipe away every tear in an instant. He is also able to walk with us through the valley of the shadow of death. We must realize that His thoughts are not our thoughts and our ways are not the same as His ways. (Is. 55:8) In this line of thought, we are able to ask our Father what our next step is. In essence, let us ask God how He wants us to best care for and repair our body and His temple (1 Cor. 6:19)

The father of lies has led us to believe the notion that if we pray and something doesn't immediately happen, then it is not God's will or God is not listening. We should not place our expectations on God. We should come before Him with gladness and praise and seek His face. We should make our request known to him. And allow him to answer as he sees fit. We need to relearn the lesson of Job. Who are we to tell God what and how to answer? Is God our servant? Should He respond as soon as we ask? Should He do as we command? Perhaps it is our pride and arrogance that leads to unanswered prayers for healing. We need to ponder this. And change the way we think.

"Praise the Lord, my soul, and forget not all His benefits – who forgives all your sins and heals all your diseases, who redeems your life from the pit and crowns you with love and compassion," (Ps. 103:2-4). We can all agree that God forgives all our sins through the blood of Jesus and redeems our life from the pit by the blood of Jesus. But why not agree with the middle segment of this scripture, that God heals all our diseases through the blood of Jesus? Later in the same psalm, David states, "as far as the east is from the west, so far has he removed our transgressions from us." (Ps. 103:12). God has separated our sin from us, as far as the east is from the west. We believe this and praise God for it because His word says it. Let's also hear and believe that He heals all our diseases.

"What do you think?"

Matthew 21:28

1. What is your belief on what the Scriptures say about physical healing?

2. Why do you think there is much debate and various interpretations on praying for healing?

Go Deeper

Luke 15:11-32
Isaiah 53:5
Malachi 3:6
James 5:14-16
Jeremiah 30:17

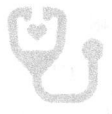

CHAPTER 3

Testimony of
Delayed Healing

---

*"So in everything, do to others
what you would have them do
to you, for this sums up the
Law and the Prophets."*

Matthew 7:12

One afternoon, my wife and I were standing in line at a local gas station with our favorite coffees in hand. We were on our way to a college baseball game and were not particularly in the mind of spiritual matters. A well dressed, athletic gentleman came up to me and shook my hand enthusiastically. As he smiled, he danced a little number in front of us. I'm sure I had this mixed look of amusement and confusion. He said, "You don't remember me, do you?"

"No sir, I don't! What is your name? How do I know you?" I replied. He asked, "You are the pharmacist, right? You prayed for my foot, remember?"

A few months back, he slowly hobbled into the pharmacy and plopped down on a waiting area chair. He was experiencing ankle pain from a work-related injury and needed a brace and supportive meds for a terrible foot sprain. I remember our pharmacy technician asking him what happened. When the technician looked at me, we instantly received the same message from the Holy Spirit.

"Go."

We walked out to the waiting area, and after a brief interchange of informative facts about his leg, asked if we could pray for him. He nodded in the affirmative through his mask. We bent down and placed our hands on his ankle and began to pray for God's healing to come to his ankle and declared God's word to that ankle.

We both proclaimed that ankle was fearfully and wonderfully made. God knit him together in his mother's womb. God's word says if two agree, He will answer. God's word says we have been given authority to use His name. Jesus said we would do what He did and more. Isaiah said that by Jesus' stripes this ankle is healed. We commanded the bones, tendons, ligaments, and muscles to line up with the word of God. The man joined in and spoke healing in the name of Jesus. When we finished, he looked unchanged physically. He nodded his thanks as the technician and I exchanged looks that asked, "Did we get that right, because nothing happened?" In due course, the man left with his brace and medications.

Now, as I stared in amazement at his fully recovered ankle at the gas station, he said that our prayers made a notable difference in his healing. "I have never had a doctor, nurse, nobody like that, offer to pray for me, a perfect stranger. But y'all got on your knees and prayed for me. That did something to me inside. I was struggling on the inside, and your prayer made me realize that others care and that God sees me." He slipped me a $20 bill to pay for our coffees. He clasped my hands closed around that $20 bill over my objections. I realized he was blessing me now. I thanked him, and we all thanked our Good Father together.

Looking back, he did not jump up from the chair with walking and leaping and praising God. Rather, there were some awkward moments for him and for us. We were being obedient to God's leading, and that's all that mattered. We prayed, and then the results were not up to us. He hobbled out of the store and out of sight. This is a picture of how many prayer sessions go. We pray and then go on with our day.

Rarely does someone stand up straight and proclaim, "I am healed!" This teaches us obedience in faith. We walk by faith and not by sight. We pray as Jesus commanded. Then, the entire matter is in the Master's Hands. His ways are higher than ours. We may think we are praying for healing of an ankle, but what we may really be doing is activating someone's faith in the goodness of God. The healing is a side benefit of the bigger picture God has planned.

Encounters such as that demand some contemplation and thought after the fact. Where was God in the story? Who was God speaking to at the pharmacy? What was God trying to accomplish in him? In me? In our technician? I did not know God was working on him prior to his visit to my pharmacy. He didn't expect someone of another race to come around the counter, bend down in front of him in a servant's position, and attend to his ailment. However, God healed his foot. And his heart wound.

How often do we pass by opportunities to be doers of the word and not hearers only? If the situation is awkward or stretches you out of your comfort zone, it is likely the Holy Spirit nudging you into a new area of growth. Fear and preconceived expectations of the unknown give us pause and oftentimes prevent us from being the hands of Jesus.

God blessed my wife and me with free coffee, and a bear claw (maybe I should have gotten two!). The main beneficiary was God! All glory to Him! What a privilege to be a tool in the Master's hand and be used to repair one of his beloved sons. There is joy unspeakable in that. Our culture might want us to think, if we pray and the person does not jump up and run laps around the building, that we are a failure, God is a fraud, and you look ridiculous in front of everyone. However, if we are obedient and can ignore the doubts in our minds and focus on God's word, we will see God work like only He can.

"What do you think?"

Matthew 21:28

1. Can you think of a time that you felt the nudge to pray for someone but did not? What were your feelings during the prompting? What were your feelings after the opportunity passed?

2. How can you grow from your experience in the previous question?

Go Deeper

James 1:22
Matthew 10:8
Galatians 5:13
1 Corinthians 15:58
Matthew 5:16

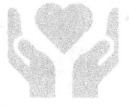

CHAPTER 4

Set The Tone in Your Workspace

"Truly I tell you, whatever you bind
on earth will be bound in heaven,
and whatever you loose on earth
will be loosed in heaven."

Matthew 18:18

Whether you are a healthcare provider in a large multiplex hospital, a physical therapy clinic, a cozy dental office, or a busy pharmacy, that is your workspace. Take a look around your workspace. You have organized and situated all of the rooms as you would like them, from the aesthetics to functionality. Your design fingerprints are seen everywhere. From the consent forms in the clipboards, to the trash can placements, to the chairs in the lobby, you are familiar with this space and comfortable in it.

My seventh grade English Teacher set the tone in his classroom. He was foreboding, stern, and a disciplinarian. He would stand in the middle of the hallway and direct traffic, "Stay to the right!' His classroom was set up like all the other teachers in our grade. However, there was a distinct aura present in his room. His lessons were given in silence. I can still hear the bottoms of his penny loafers scratch the floor as he whirled around to catch the offender of the class rules. He demanded discipline. He demanded effort. Those of us who gave effort and adhered to his discipline learned English proficiently. I promise you that my freshman English class in college was merely a review of his concepts.

In a similar manner, you set the tone in your workspace. Why not set up your workspace in the Spirit of God? Your workspace should have a distinct aura. You should work to cultivate an atmosphere of love and joy and peace. All sorts of patients come to your workplace with many types of moods and dispositions. These are evident in the expression on their faces and the evidence of body language. Fear. Anxiety. Hate. Unworthiness. Orphan Mentality. Suicidality. Rage. Confusion.

"All scripture is God-breathed and is useful for teaching, rebuking, correcting and training in righteousness, so that the servant of God may be thoroughly equipped for every good work." (2 Tim. 3:16-17). From The Passion Translation, those same verses are, "God has transmitted His very substance into every Scripture, for it is God-breathed. It will empower you by its instruction and correction, giving you strength to take the right direction and lead you deeper into the path of Godliness. Then you will be God's servant, fully mature and perfectly prepared to fulfill any assignment God gives you."

One of the many fundamental truths in these familiar verses is the idea that God's word is so complex and deep and wide that it applies to every facet of our lives. God breathed life into us. As His breath is in our lungs, so is His breath in His Word. It is a living document.

Through this lens, there are many Scriptures that we can apply to our workspace so that we "may be thoroughly equipped for every good work." Please do not discount this word. The verse does not say somewhat equipped for very specific works only. The verse does not even imply that God's word is only in effect when presenting the gospel to the heathen. This verse says, "for every good work." As a healthcare worker, you are doing "good work." You are helping the Lord Jesus provide life more abundantly. So, let's apply His word, His breath of life, to our workplace.

Matthew 18:18, "Truly I tell you, whatever you bind on earth will be bound in heaven and whatever you loose on earth will be loosed in heaven." Your patients are influenced by their feelings and preconceptions of you who are and the type of care they will receive. Many patients come into your workplace with negative attitudes with which they freely inoculate everyone nearby. While we must be compassionate and empathetic to all patients, we must also create an environment conducive to the flow of the Spirit of the Lord.

Take charge of your rooms. Speak with authority given to you as a Believer into the room. Bind up the spirits of profanity, anger, rage... you fill in the blank. For some of you practitioners with a bunch of starch in your collar, this may be foreign to you or seem out of the scope of what Jesus permits us to do. This scripture gives us permission to bind these negative influences and forbid their expression and actions in our presence. An essential follow-up is to loose "shalom peace" into the room. Ask the Father to send His angels into your rooms with the peace of heaven. When you pray this out loud and with authority, you will sense the atmosphere of the room shift.

"You, dear children, are from God and have overcome them, because the one who is in you is greater than the one who is in the world." (1 Jn. 4:4). The NLT version reads: "But you belong to God, my dear children. You have already won a victory over those people, because the Spirit who lives in you is greater than the spirit who lives in the world."

"So God created mankind in his own image, in the image of God he created them; male and female he created them. God blessed them and said to them, 'Be fruitful and increase in number; fill the earth and subdue it.'" (Gen. 1:27-28a). Father God created us to reign. We are in charge. Do not forfeit your responsibility or authority to any negative influence or manifesting demonic behavior. "I will give you every place where you set your foot, as I promised Moses." (Josh. 1:3). Your office workspace is your land.

After "praying up" the room, reign with humble authority. "For we are God's handiwork, created in Christ Jesus to do good works, which God prepared in advance for us to do" (Eph. 2:10). To draw on the NLT version again," For we are God's masterpiece. He has created us anew in Christ Jesus, so we can do the good things He planned for us long ago." God has placed you in that room to help His children take their next step toward the abundant life.

"But the fruit of the Spirit is love, joy, peace, patience, kindness, goodness, faithfulness, gentleness and self control. There is no law against these things!" (Gal. 5:22-23). Pray these upon yourself on the way to work. Realize that patients come into your office hurting, don't feel well, and probably are not in a great mood. The patient doesn't need you to bark back when he barks first. Instead, give out peace and patience. You shift the atmosphere. Turn the other cheek and instead bless them with a genuine smile and kindness and self-control. Prepare in advance for the negative emotions and pledge that you will return a basketful of Spiritual fruit instead.

"Therefore, put on the full armor of God, so that when the day of evil comes, you may be able to stand your ground, and after you have done everything, to stand." (Eph 6:13) This is another excellent prayer to pray over yourself. The attacks of the enemy come in various forms, and you have been given armor to protect you and help you stand firm.

Consider these and many other scriptures as you prepare your work environment in such a way that you will naturally be a doer of the Word and not a hearer only. (Jam. 1:2 NKJV).

"Commit your actions to the Lord, and your plans will succeed." (Prov. 16:3 NLT)

"Yet I am always with you; you hold me by my right hand. You guide me with your counsel…" (Ps. 73:23-24)

"Be strong and courageous. Do not be afraid or terrified because of them, for the Lord your God goes with you; He will never leave you nor forsake you." (Deut. 31:6)

"For this reason I remind you to fan into flame the gift of God, which is in you through the laying on of my hands. For the Spirit God gave us does not make us timid, but gives us power, love and self-discipline." (2 Tim. 1:6-7)

The NKJV puts it better in some ways: "Therefore I remind you to stir up the gift of God which is in you through the laying on of my hands. For God has not given us a spirit of fear, but of power and of love and of a sound mind." (2 Tim. 1:6-7)

"But one who prophesies strengthens others, encourages them, and comforts them." (1 Cor. 14:3)

"What do you think?"

Matthew 21:28

1. How has this chapter prepared you to prepare your workplace for prayer?

2. What hindrances do you foresee in equipping your workplace for prayer?

Go Deeper

Joshua 1:3
Deut 31:6
Isaiah 55:11
Luke 10:5
Rev 12:11

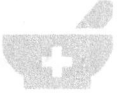

CHAPTER 5

Pray For the Caregivers

"And we know that in all things God works for the good of those who love Him, who have been called according to his purpose."

Romans 8:28

A defining moment for me in praying for patients occurred when the husband of a hospice patient came into the pharmacy one day with a stern but concerned look on his face. His look asked many questions. What will I do as a single parent with 2 teenagers? Why is this happening to my wife? Have we exhausted all possible remedies? Am I dreaming?

I knew from her profile that the patient was in her early 40's. Facial cancer was the diagnosis. The husband carried an edge to him that warned if any slight detail were off, he may explode. When I saw him come in, I sensed my spirit quicken and my body tense a bit. But I knew I must talk to him. "Hi, Lucas," I began. No need to flash my grin and ask him how he was doing. His countenance told me all that I needed to know.

"How is Debbie doing today?" His stone jaw turned away slightly and clinched as if to stifle the tear. He shook his head in the negative. At this point, I motioned for him to meet me at the consultation window. He leaned in with his elbows on the counter but his head slumped to his chest. This proud and self-reliant man had come up against something that brute strength or cunning intelligence could not conquer. "I hate this, man." He began to shake his head rhythmically and slowly in the negative. When he looked up, the red in his watery eyes detailed the pain he was experiencing.

This is a crucial time. Any flippant word or joke or any medical stats or fanatical preaching would damage him deeply. So I just empathetically looked at him, ready to listen to anything he wanted to say. Romans 12:15 instructs us to, "Rejoice with those who rejoice, and weep with those who weep." (NKJV)

Lucas pulled out his cell phone and showed me a picture of Debbie's face. The entire picture was of her grossly inflamed cheek area from just below the eyes and down to the chin. At about where cute dimples should have been, a bulge of what looked like Playdoh protruded outwardly and even distorted her lip. What do you say at this point? Lucas has just gotten extremely vulnerable really quickly. His command was succinct, "Look."

"Do you mind if I pray for you?" I asked. He lowered the phone and stared at me with his swollen blue eyes. His stare attempted to bore straight through me. His eyes asked, "What good would it do?" He nodded in the affirmative anyway, and I asked for his hand. He gripped my hand firmly but never looked away. I sensed now was not the time for a long-winded prayer.

I asked God to dwell in the midst of this issue with him and his family. For shalom peace to cover him from the top of his head to the soles of his feet. To know that You are near, Father. Without the traditional "amen", I asked if I could pray for Debbie. When he nodded yes, I asked him to pull up that picture and let's both put our hands on it. I basically prayed the same prayer for Debbie. I did not get the leading from the Spirit to pray for supernatural complete healing. Perhaps I missed it. However, the peace that drifted into the patient consult area was proof that the prayer was appropriate and heard.

I am one of the weird guys that checks the obituaries online in our local newspaper. Debbie's name never appeared. A week later, Lucas came into the pharmacy. He smiled, then nodded at me and told me he was moving back to Florida. Debbie passed peacefully two days ago. He thanked me for taking time with him and that he would never forget it.

Then, the sentinel moment happened. Lucas turned his head slightly in an inquisitive fashion and asked, "You're more than a pharmacist, aren't you? Are you a preacher?" It was time to stand up and be counted. I shall stand

and declare who I am. After a deep breath and realizing that several people turned to listen to my reply, I confidently said, "I am a disciple of Jesus. Each day, I want to get to know Him better, become like Him and do what He did." Then, I exhaled with relief for some reason. Lucas stopped and that rock solid stare that he flashed the first time we met returned. "Keep up the good work," he said with a slight smile and walked out of the store.

Over the next month, I tried to connect with Lucas several times. The phone number I had for him was invalid, and Debbie's was turned off. I have not seen him since, but I prayed for him occasionally as the days went by. Here is a man who was cut deeply by the enemy, and I prayed that he did not blame God. I also prayed that he would experience the complete love of the Father.

Being willing to pray for patients often takes us to places that we do not expect. For Lucas, I suspect he was presented with a version of "religion" that was new to him and got him thinking. For me, that experience solidified my role as a praying pharmacist. No turning back.

"What do you think?"

Matthew 21:28

1. What are the unique needs of the caregiver? Consider the various types of patient needs, from post operative care to long term disability.

2. What key ingredient is needed to pray for the caregiver instead of the patient?

Go Deeper

Luke 10:30-35
Ruth 1:16-17
Esther 4:14
Hebrews 6:10
Matthew 5:16

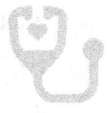

CHAPTER 6

Prayer Helps the Practitioner

"Come to me, all you who are
weary and burdened, and I
will give you rest."

Matthew 11:28

Merriam-Webster defines burnout in the occupational sense as "exhaustion of physical or emotional strength or motivation usually as a result of prolonged stress or frustration." Even a casual examination of this definition leads the reader to see the key points.

First is "exhaustion of physical or emotional strength or motivation". We get tired of the same-old, same-old. Whether it's filling thousands of prescriptions for metformin or looking into thousands of pediatric ears, we all reach a point of exhaustion. Constant pressure to perform, which is fueled by our desire to serve others and see them well, begins to wear bald spots on our tires. A brilliant pediatrician friend of mine calls this "brain atrophy." As a protectant, we go into auto-pilot. We cannot muster the same intensity and carry the same energy as we once did. We are exhausted.

Secondly, "…usually as a result of pro-longed stress or frustration." Anything that provides prolonged stress or frustration can lead to burnout. Jesus told us to come to Him, "all you who labor and are heavy laden, and I will give you rest." (Matt. 11:28 NKJV) Jesus gives us rest.

Have you ever sat in His presence and experienced His peace that passes all under-standing? It is rather easy to do. God is every-where. He is behind the curtain in ICU. He is sitting in the crowded waiting area beside the mother who is holding the screaming child. He is beside me as I type this and beside you as you read this. Recognize Him. Invite Him into the situation. Feel the tension and the frustration give way to the peace of the Lord.

Many times, even in our church services, we believe music is a must to worship the Lord. If we are not careful, we will spend most of our time reading the words off the screen and trying to keep in time musically rather than connect with the Father. "I will praise the Lord at all times; His praise will always be on my lips." (Ps. 34:1 HCSB) I encourage you to begin to speak out your praise to the Lord in much the same way as you would speak into the drive-thru speaker at the local hamburger joint. Learn to do this without music and without singing. Speak the goodness of God and repeat His blessings in His Scriptures over your life.

Here are a few examples. I am fearfully and wonderfully made. The Lord is my Shepherd, and I lack nothing. He will never leave me nor forsake me. The Lord guides me by my right hand. He fills my cup to overflowing. He prepares a table for me in the presence of my enemies. His goodness and mercy follow me everyday. The Lord has no rival or equal. He is incomparable. Nothing slips His mind. He misses no detail. He even knows the very number of hairs in my life.

There are so many promises in the Scriptures that we can speak over our lives and into the places where we live, work, and visit. Read the Psalms and other scriptures of praise. Repeat those blessings and wonderful attributes about our Father back to Him. Father God loves to hear his kids praise Him. He smiles at us with the warmest and proudest of smiles! Develop your praise language. Speak into your work environment those praises that you love to say and that God loves to hear. Be thankful unto Him and bless His name!

It is vital to understand that doing this helps us as practitioners. Each day, we face 10-12 hours or more of multi-tasking which provide varying degrees of difficulties and severity. These situations may involve trauma patients struggling for their next breath, anxious teenagers consumed with social media pressures, arguments over co-pays and other financial matters, or even superiors who do not understand your stress and demand more production.

Praying for a patient allows us to jump off the speeding train and focus on one individual. All else sinks into the background. Mark 10:46-52 gives us a picture of this. Jesus is on His way to Jerusalem and has predicted His death for the third time to non-understanding followers who have been with Him for three years. He had to endure these same twelve debating who will sit where in the Kingdom of Heaven, without any hint of comprehension that Jesus will be put to death soon. When they enter Jericho, they encounter a blind man who intentionally seeks out the Lord Jesus. He is persistent in his cries to Jesus. And Jesus stops. Jesus became a servant to the blind man. Verse 51 states, "What do you want me to do for you?"

Jesus is asking us to become a servant to those in need. Sure, our patients need our training, expertise, and sound medical judgements. They also need our compassion and kindness. When we stop to pray for our patient, this pulls us out of the hecticness and sets us in a one-on-one Divine Appointment. This provides palpable physical and spiritual energy to the Praying Practitioner. It breaks up the nonstop routines and chaos and allows us to look at the Author and Finisher of our faith. He is the One who is the same yesterday, today and forevermore. As we pray for our patient, our strength increases, our faith rises, and our smiles come back.

All you need is to see one patient positively impacted by prayer and you will not stop praying thereafter.

"What do you think?"

Matthew 21:28

1. What activities have you tried in an attempt to prevent work-related burnout?

2. What do you think about the Divine Appointment concept?

Go Deeper

Deut 1:26
John 4:4
John 6:8
Acts 9:11-12
Acts 10:20,

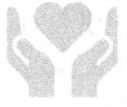

CHAPTER 7

Healing Blocked Until Forgiveness Was Granted

"For if you forgive other people when they sin against you, your heavenly Father will also forgive you."

Matthew 6:14

A long-time patient of ours came to the pharmacy with a prescription for a muscle relaxer. As we began to chat, she mentioned that both of her legs have been hurting for a while. She went on to relate that her doctor has done tests and cannot pinpoint the problem, as the x-ray and MRI have come back unremarkable.

This was when my Holy Spirit radar began pinging. This was a spiritual issue. In this instance, the first step is to determine if the patient can identify the exact day or event when the pain started. "Gloria, I believe this pain has a spiritual origin. Are you willing to talk about that possibility?" She nodded yes, but I could see in her eyes she already knew where this was going and was debating whether or not she wanted to get back into that painful memory. This would require recalling and describing events that she had suppressed because of the agony.

I recognized this look and asked the question again. I did not want to force her into a place that she was not wanting to go. She sniffled up the courage and nodded faster this time. "Yes" was her only verbal reply.

No need to beat the rug too long. "When exactly did this pain start?" Gloria replied, "When I climbed up into my husband's jacked up truck one day, cramps grabbed both of my legs and they have not been the same since." Of course, she had jumped up in this truck numerous times before, but this particular time was different. This was the physical movement she was making when the pain started, but this was not what was happening spiritually. "What was going on that day or during that time in your life?"

A reliable clue that you have hit the tender spot is the evidence of speaking in tears. Her eyes moistened rapidly and she glanced away. I stood there patiently but kept silently kept eye contact.

"My daughter..." Gloria's abdomen racked and she inhaled deeply with a choppy wheeze. "She was sexually assaulted by someone we trusted... touched inappropriately... and then we were told to keep quiet to keep God's blessings flowing in our lives."

Um, Holy Spirit, I really, really need You right now. My usual disposition is one of light-heartedness. I often have a joke or quip to lighten the mood when facing heavy conversation, but there was no place for such things at this moment. I stood there in silence, praying rapidly in my mind for the Holy Spirit to take charge of my tongue and say what He wanted to say. Gloria had opened up the clam shell of her soul to expose the hidden, dark secret to me.

By this time, we moved to a private location where she felt safe enough to talk without being overheard. My mouth opened and said, "It's okay to tell God how you feel. It's scriptural. Psalm 142 is proof." Gloria nodded and shared that she has hollered and screamed to God about the issue while alone. She said that, after that event, her daughter left the church and turned to a same-sex relationship. This event drove a wedge between Gloria and her daughter. The perpetrator went on with his life as if nothing occurred.

"Gloria, do you know what your next step is in this situation to obtain freedom?" She just stared at me. Her eyes said that she could not. Would not. "When you are ready, you must forgive him. Completely. This is the critical step to healing." Tears made their way over the crest of her cheek and down towards her chin. Pain was leaving. The Spirit was ministering, loving and touching her. She began to slowly rock back and forth, followed by a faster rock of the head.

"I am not rushing you. I cannot imagine the pain. But Jesus is willing to take all of those feelings if you put them on a plate and give them to Him. He will not take them from you. You must surrender them to Him." I left her at the table to attend to a few phone calls and prescriptions.

A few minutes later, I noticed Gloria walking up and down the aisles of the pharmacy. She seemed to be talking to herself, or perhaps to the Father.

Jesus has already paid for all of it in full. So render unto Caesar what is Caesar's and to Jesus what is Jesus's. Since He paid for the sin, give it to Him. He wants it because He paid for it. Why are we holding onto it? Give it to the rightful owner. Then, taste and see what Jesus will give you in return!

In Gloria's case, I noticed her health dwindling over the course of the last few years. I believe this spiritual situation was the root cause of her physical suffering. Once the root cause was dealt with appropriately, she would be on her way to healing.

I found her amongst the OTC eye products. "Gloria, thank you for opening up and sharing.

I believe we both know the next step, and when you are ready, I would be happy to lead you through it with the help of the Lord."

"Let's do it now."

The Scriptures tell us several key principles to guide us at this point. "Confess your sins to each other and pray for each other so that you may be healed." (James 5:16). "Bear with each other and forgive one another if any of you has a grievance against someone. Forgive as the Lord forgave you." (Col 3:13) A growing body of evidence, even in the non-evangelical scientific community, has noted forgiveness of others and releasing grudges is related to increased overall health measures. Do not underestimate the power of forgiving others who have wronged the patient, which in turn leads to that patient's healing. God's word does not return void. (Is. 55). Forgiveness is very important to the Father.

I led Gloria through a series of short, declarative statements. She proclaimed aloud that she chose to forgive the perpetrator completely (she mentioned his name as I plugged my ears). She forgave herself for her involvement.

Then she canceled any agreements with darkness over this issue and commanded the pain to leave in the name of Jesus!

Gloria walked around and said her legs were already feeling better! I encouraged her to proclaim the goodness of God and praise His name. Some breakthroughs are gradual, and some are immediate. However, all of them need support and nurturing. I invited her and her daughter to our church. She left the pharmacy a different person than what she was when she entered. Whom the Son sets free is free indeed! (Jn. 8:36)

"What do you think?"

Matthew 21:28

1. What are your thoughts or experiences with the connection of forgiveness and healing?

2. How can you encourage your patients to forgive or seek forgiveness?

Go Deeper

Leviticus 26:1-6
1 John 1:9
Psalm 103:12
Luke 17:4
Ephesians 4:3

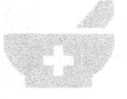

CHAPTER 8

When The Answer Is Not What We Want and It Hurts

"The secret things belong to the
Lord our God, but the things
revealed belong to us and to our
children forever, that we may
follow all the words of this law."

Deuteronomy 29:29

Years ago, my wife and I attended a church in which there was a young boy stricken with bone cancer. He was only 7 years old and such a sweet and happy child. The urge to pray for Spencer arose in our church to the point where the announcement was made from the pulpit to meet on a particular night to intercede for Spencer. Over a hundred people came to pray that night! Spencer, his mom, and dad stayed in the church while all the attendees slowly walked around the church. This was to encircle the family in prayer and call on God for a miracle. Some read Scriptures aloud and knelt to pray during the hour of prayer.

During my slow walk counterclockwise around the church, I could sense the presence of Father God. It was as if an electric force field was emanating from the church building. I also thought I heard the humming buzz of electricity. This was not a fearful presence but rather an intensely focused presence. Many were weeping and some stopped in silence. Such an intense corporate prayer for healing arose from those church grounds that night!

At the end of the hour, my wife and I drove home, mostly in silence. We both agreed that surely, the presence of the Lord was there. Surely, we would hear the evidence of a miracle. Surely, the Lord touched Spencer that night and he was healed. What an amazing testimony he would be! We could envision him going on into ministry to intercede and encourage others in a similar situation.

A few weeks later our congregation sat in silence as the pastor related the heartbreaking news that Spencer went home to be with the Lord the previous night. The only ambient sound was that of the HVAC system humming. What does one say now? Do now? How do we react to this news as professing and believing Christians? Am I now in a faith struggle? Has my level of faith in God decreased? What will be my attitude and disposition the next time someone wants prayer?

Romans 12:15 instructs us to, "Weep with those who weep." NKJV). Nowhere in the Greek does this verse read, "weep and try to explain why the prayer was not answered because this will help the parents who just lost their child." Oftentimes, it is simply your silent presence that is the most comforting during times of loss. The less you speak verbally, the more you will speak from the heart.

We must understand that Satan hates us. We are made in the image of God. From the beginning, we were all created and designed to reign with God over angels, which includes Satan. Hebrews 1:14 asks the question, "Are not all angels ministering spirits sent to serve those who will inherit salvation?" Lucifer was one of those angels, and he did not want to serve humans. This issue was a cornerstone of his rebellion. As a result, he wages war on those who are made in the image of God Almighty. Disease and trauma come as a result of the curse pursuant to our disobedience. Satan gladly spills his bowl of diseases over humanity. Whether or not we choose to acknowledge this is irrelevant. It is the fact of our reality.

The heartbreaking reality is that sometimes our patients die anyway. During these times, the enemy loves to stop by and smoke a cigarette while staring with a grin. The enemy attacks us in our thought life. This is a fundamental reason to continually meditate on the scriptures. If we have God's words in our minds, there is little room for the enemy. It is written: "Submit yourselves, then, to God. Resist the devil, and he will flee from you. Come near to God and He will come near to you." (James 4:7-8a).

Some have mentioned that our prayer for Spencer was unanswered. How do we define "unanswered?" Is an unanswered prayer one whose outcome is different than what we envisioned? This has been my opinion in certain experiences. But the question remains, was the prayer "unanswered," or was it answered with a "no"?

By no means do I have God's Top 10 Reasons for not answering prayer in the manner I wish. However, there are some basic realities that I have noticed over the years that prevent God from moving in the direction He naturally wants. These are incorporated into the next chapter on hindrances to prayer.

"What do you think?"

Matthew 21:28

1. What has been your response internally and externally to unanswered prayer, or prayer answered with a no?

2. How have you responded to a patient for whom you prayed for healing and the healing has not occurred yet?

Go Deeper

Luke 18:1-8
Isaiah 55:8-9
Deuteronomy 30:15-20
Job 11:7-10
Habakkuk 3:17-19

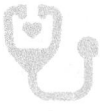

CHAPTER 9

Our Hindrances to Prayer

"Let us not become weary in doing good, for at the proper time we will reap a harvest if we do not give up."

Galatians 6:9

The devil will try to convince us not to pray for our patients. The primary attack on us occurs between our ears. The weapons the enemy uses to prevent us from initiating prayer for our patients are fear, doubt, and nervousness to engage. The enemy also uses temptations to lure us away or distract us from praying.

We face the temptation to quit praying when results are not seen after praying for our patients. We face the temptation to dismiss the unction to go pray in the name of not having time to pray. We face the temptation to rationalize that we are physicians, pharmacologists, and therapists, and we know the data of the patient's disease and nothing changes that scientifically.

The alternate temptations are just as dangerous. Let me at 'em. I am on a roll. The last 4 people I prayed for gave me instant feedback that they felt better, and their physical exams confirmed the healings. So, we pray for patients without God's leading and blessing, and we fall flat. Then doubt creeps into our minds.

How do we combat these hindrances? We overcome them with the word of God. How did Jesus combat temptation from the devil? He did not mince words. He quoted the Word of God with authority and faith. As a Praying Practitioner, it is vital that you memorize at least a few verses regarding the subject of physical healing. Please refer to the Go Deeper section at the end of this chapter for a few suggestions. These scriptures are a sharp two-edged sword that is a weapon against the lies of the enemy. (Heb. 4:11)

A hindrance typically observed on the part of a patient is the excuse, "It is not God's will that I be healed." If this is your belief, go ahead and ask God to make you as miserable and disease ridden as possible. Sounds ridiculous doesn't it? "He who did not spare His own Son, but gave him up for us all – how will he not also, along with him, graciously give us all things?" (Rom. 8:32). Overall, it is His will that His children have life, and that more abundantly, and live to a good old age. (Jn. 10:10; Gen. 15:15). I do not believe it is God's sovereign will for anyone to die before the good old age is reached, or for anyone to die of disease. I believe this is one of the reasons Jesus commands us to "raise the dead." (Matt. 10:8). People need a chance to live an abundant, full life.

Another hindrance is found in the accusation that, "God is punishing me with this disease." Our Father in heaven is a good Father (Ps. 100:5) who delights in His children (Zeph. 3:17) and knows how to give good gifts (Lk.

11:13). Allow me to use that previous paragraph's logic on you. If you were upset with your child and wanted to teach her a lesson, would you curse her with a disease? Of course not. This idea that God is punishing me with this disease is totally out to lunch. It is a lie from the pit of hell. God so loved us that He gave us His ONLY begotten Son. So, flush this idea that disease is punishment from the loving Father.

The last hindrance I want to address is, "I hope I will be healed one day." This desperate cry lacks any sort of asking or receiving from the Father. This line of thought is an avenue that many take to give up and resign oneself to a life of disease. It is analogous to saying, "I hope I will be saved one day."

None of us, who have asked Jesus to be Lord of our life, says, "I hope Jesus will save me." Hope is future tense. We must stop hoping for something that is already ours. Healing is the children's bread, given to them by their heavenly Father, (Matt. 15:26).

Many evangelists over the years have declared that faith is an action verb. Faith is now.

We receive by acting in faith on the authority given to us by the shed blood of Jesus Christ of Nazareth. "Therefore, I tell you, whatever you ask for in prayer, believe that you have received it, and it will be yours." (Mk. 11:24). Even when the situation looks bleak, continue to believe in faith (now) for the healing touch of the Father.

Proverbs 18:21 says "death and life are in the power of the tongue, and those who love it will eat its fruit." (NKJV). Another ending of that verse from the NLT is "those who love to talk will reap the consequences." It is imperative to get our patients to begin to speak positives over their lives. Consider preparing 5 verses on a card to give to patients who need a positive word in their lives.

Remind the patients that they are fearfully and wonderfully made. God knit them together in their mother's womb. God takes delight in them. They are the apple of God's eye. Our Father in heaven gave His only begotten Son for your patients. There are many more encouraging verses in the Bible. Select the ones that resonate with you and that will impact your patients positively.

Develop the discernment necessary to be sensitive to the leading of Holy Spirit. Sometimes, Holy Spirit does not lead you to pray for someone at that time. One example occurs in Acts. "Now a man who was lame from birth was being carried to the temple gate called Beautiful, where he was put every day to beg from those going into the temple courts." (Acts 3:2). The Lord Jesus surely passed this man on the way into the temple mount numerous times. However, it was two of His disciples upon whom the unction came to command this man's healing, and this was not until after Jesus' ascension to heaven.

It is critical to understand that this is not an escape clause to avoid praying for our patients. Even when we are not praying with a patient, we should be praying for that patient. It is a matter of divine timing. "There is a time for everything, and a season for every activity under the heavens." (Ecc. 3:1). Sometimes, the ground must be tilled several times before a seed is planted. There will come a time, however, that the Father will orchestrate, in which the patient is ready to receive the prayer of faith. This is when the undeniable prompting of Holy Spirit will occur. At that moment, open your mouth and allow Holy Spirit to speak to your patient.

"What do you think?"

Matthew 21:28

1. What is your primary reason for hesitation or your main hindrance that stops you from praying for your patients?

2. What can you do to overcome this hesitation or hindrance?

Go Deeper

Isaiah 53:5
Proverbs 4:20-22
Romans 8:32
Jeremiah 30:17
2 Chronicles 30:20

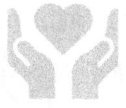

CHAPTER 10

When The Patient Does Not Want Prayer

"Then the people began to plead with Jesus to leave their region."

Mark 5:17

Some patients do not want prayer. For whatever reason, prayer is not an option for them. If you decide to ask a patient if you may pray for them, and they say no, this could turn into an awkward moment unless you are prepared to hear no. This chapter discusses some of the reasons that you may hear no, as well as what to do when you hear no. It is critical to the spirit of the Praying Practitioner not to take the "no" personally or offensively.

A popular reason you may receive a "no" to your invitation to pray is that the patient has observed your lifestyle. "If anyone thinks they are something when they are not, they deceive themselves." (Gal 6:3). People notice your walk and your talk. When you claim to be a Christian, you have officially invited microscopic scrutiny of your life. Patients will want to know that you are genuine before they become vulnerable with you. Do you actually walk out what you talk about?

If your lifestyle does not match your Christian words, do not be surprised when patients roll their eyes and frown when you ask them if you may pray for them. As Jesus said, by their fruit you will recognize them. It is imperative that you live a life that displays evidence of you pursuing God. We cannot give away what we do not have.

Another reason a patient may decline your prayer request is if they feel like you are forcing something on them. Most people can tell when you begin to apply pressure to them to convert their way of thinking or change their behavior about a particular subject. If you get the impression nonverbally that the patient is resistant to prayer, it is best not to push the subject. A little salt on the cucumber slice tastes great. A big pile of salt on the slice of cucumber is nauseating.

When we do make the offer to pray, if the patient declines, we should honor that decision. Whether or not we feel like we are the next Smith Wigglesworth is irrelevant. If the patient wanted prayer, he or she would have agreed to receive prayer.

Some of our patients do not believe in any God. We understand the fact that God so loved them that He sent His only Son into the world. We understand that while they were yet sinners, Christ died for our patients. We understand that they are made in the image of God. Our task is to help the Holy Spirit generate a hunger in them for more of the Father. Thus, one of the best things we can give them the love of the Father.

A common argument from atheists regarding praying for healing is that it is not a 100% return on investment. Sometimes we pray and patients get better, and sometimes they do not recover. This is seen as random chance to the atheist. If you meet a feisty atheist who wants to debate you and become antagonistic, it is best to turn the cheek and smile. As the proverb goes, whoever corrects a mocker invites insult. (Prov. 9:7). However, lift up a prayer to God Almighty for that patient later in the day outside of their presence. Ask Holy Spirit to soften their hearts so they will realize that God is good and that He desires a relationship with them.

For some people, previous prayers that were unanswered according to the pray-er's preference have led them to believe that God is not interested in them. Thus, they become uninterested in the things of God. These patients believe the lie that satan whispers to them: "God doesn't care about you." Unfortunately, these persons do not want prayer. With these patients, avoid the bait of the enemy to provide a list of plausible explanations as to why previous prayers were unfulfilled. Now is the time to give away the fruit of the Spirit. Kindness and gentleness are the prescriptions needed at this time. It is the Holy Spirit's job to convict and deal with their hearts. It is our job to hear and understand them in love.

The last group discussed here are those who have been hurt by the church or by someone who claimed to represent God. Abuses by the church span all denominations and have resulted in cynicism or even anger toward the things of God. These patients need a touch from God and not excuses from us.

The best course of action is to love them with the Father's love. Give them the fruit of the spirit and continue to be consistent in where you stand. Perhaps one day, that patient will begin to ask questions about God or vent their frustrations about past experiences. During this time of curiosity, the patient is unknowingly vulnerable to receiving a nugget of truth from you. Perhaps the love of the Father will break through the locks on their hearts to heal past hurts. You stand firm in your belief and be ready to provide a testimony as to why you believe what Father God says.

"What do you think?"

Matthew 21:28

1. What is your experience with interacting with a patient who does not want prayer? How did you handle this situation?

2. What have you learned from patients who refuse prayer? How has this impacted your mission to pray for your patients?

Go Deeper

Isaiah 43:22
Luke 6:37
Proverbs 17:9
Psalms 34:18
Psalms 147:3

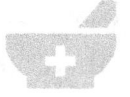

CHAPTER 11

Build Up Your Faith

"But someone will say, 'You have
faith; I have deeds.' Show me your
faith without deeds, and I will show
you my faith by my deeds."

James 2:18

Faith is believing we have something before
we can touch it or see it physically. (Heb. 11:1).
In Romans, Paul states, "If we already have
something, we don't need to hope for it." (Rom.
8:24 NLT) In that instance, we can touch and
see the item.

How did we receive salvation? It is by faith
that you are saved. (Eph. 2:8). How did we get
faith? Did we inherit it? Did we find it on the

side of the road? No. Faith comes from the breath of God. "So then faith comes by hearing, and hearing by the word of God." (Rom. 10:17 NKJV). "In the beginning was the Word, and the Word was with God, and the Word was God." (Jn. 1:1).

Faith is not an object that we place on a shelf to collect dust. Faith is an action. Every time I position myself in front of this chair to sit, I have faith that the chair will not float away, move on its own, or collapse under my weight. I just naturally assume all the variables will fall into place and this chair will hold me when I begin to sit. But I must act on this faith to sit in this chair.

Occasionally, my grandfather would give me a dollar bill when I was young. He would hold out the dollar in his calloused, oil-stained right hand. I can still see his thumb pinching that dollar bill onto his forefinger and extending the dollar toward me with a smile. I had faith that he would give the dollar to me. But I had to act on that faith to receive the dollar bill. That dollar was not mine, and neither was the pack of baseball cards that I would buy with it, until I acted in faith by reaching out, taking possession of the dollar, and bringing it to me.

What an image of our Father God in heaven! He has good things for us, but He will not cram them into our pockets. He gives us a choice. If you want it, here it is. Our Father gladly gives. "If you, then, though you are evil [we are all evil compared to Father God], know how to give good gifts to your children, how much more will your Father in heaven give good gifts to those who ask Him." (Matt. 7:11). We must act to receive the gift. Jesus said, "Here I am! I stand at the door and knock. If anyone hears my voice and opens the door, I will come in and eat with that person, and they with me." (Rev. 3:20).

Through this lens of faith requiring an action, let us consider another facet of faith. In a parable detailed in Matthew's gospel, Jesus equated acting on faith with the concept of authority. In the eighth chapter of Matthew, Jesus is approached by a centurion in Capernaum on the shores of the Sea of Galilee. The centurion is not a Jew and is considered to be an enemy. The centurion asked Jesus for help,

"... my servant lies at home paralyzed, suffering terribly." (v. 6). Jesus asked the centurion, "Shall I come and heal him?" (v. 7). The most intriguing part of this story is not that Jesus would enter the home of a sinner and defile Himself, but rather the centurion's reply.

"Lord, I do not deserve to have you come under my roof. But just say the word, and my servant will be healed." (Matt. 8:8). The centurion acted on his faith. It is apparent from this account that he knew that Jesus was Lord, that he needed to seek Jesus, and he needed to ask Jesus. I believe this was a divine setup. Jesus asked, "Shall I come heal him?" but likely had no intention of going. This was to be another lesson on faith.

The centurion stops Jesus. Can you imagine this scene? The centurion with his hand up like a traffic officer in front of Jesus, telling Him to not come to his house but to simply speak the word. The centurion explains that he understands that he himself as a centurion has authority over those who are under his command. He can speak commands, and those under his authority act accordingly. There is no question whether they will obey because the centurion has authority over them. In coming to Jesus, the centurion recognized that Jesus has this same authority over the sickness that is grievously tormenting his servant.

Amazed, Jesus equates the centurion's statements about authority with faith. "When Jesus heard this, He was amazed and said to those following Him, "Truly I tell you, I have not found anyone in Israel with such great faith." (Matt. 8:10, emphasis added). Can you imagine doing something that amazes Jesus?! "Then Jesus said to the centurion, 'Go! Let it be done just as you believed it would.' And his servant was healed at that moment." (Matt. 8:13). What is the point? Faith is applying your authority in action.

Let us turn back to the important scripture of Romans 10:17, this time in the Amplified translation. "So faith comes from hearing [what is told], and what is heard comes by the [preaching of the] message concerning Christ." This scripture tells us that when we hear the message of Christ preached, then faith comes. Let us review a few far-fetched concepts in the

Bible and see if you "believe" them or have faith in them.

"Then Moses stretched out his hand over the sea, and all that night the Lord drove the sea back with a strong east wind and turned it into dry land. The waters were divided and the Israelites went through the sea on dry ground, with a wall of water on their right and on their left." Exodus 14:21-22

Come on, now. A man stretches out his hand over the sea (the sea!) and it parts to reveal dry land?

"My God sent His angel, and he shut the mouths of the lions. They have not hurt me, because I was found innocent in his sight." Daniel 6:22

Come on, now. A man is thrown to the lions, and he chills out with them all night without a scratch?

"'You will conceive and give birth to a son, and you are to call Him Jesus. He will be great and will be called the Son of the Most High. The Lord God will give him the throne of his father David, and he will reign over Jacob's descendants forever; his kingdom will never end.'

'How will this be,' Mary asked the angel, 'since I am a virgin.'" Luke 1:31-34

Come on, now. A teenage girl will conceive and give birth to the only begotten Son of Almighty God although she is a virgin?

"When they had rowed about three or four miles, they saw Jesus approaching the boat, walking on the water; and they were frightened." John 6:19

Come on, now. No one can walk on water. Human bodies are more dense than the water, and they will sink.

"The angel said to the women, 'Do not be afraid, for I know that you are looking for Jesus, who was crucified. He is not here; he has risen, just as he said. Come and see the place where he lay.'" Matthew 28:5-6

Come on, now. A man is brutally beaten and crucified by the Romans, and he rose from the dead after 3 days?

These are commonly taught stories of the Bible. We believe them because we heard these stories preached. We have read these stories in the Bible (the Word). We have participated in children's plays that act out the various scenes we read about above. We believe them. We have faith that these events occurred because they are in the Word of God that we heard spoken to us. "All scripture is God-breathed and is useful for teaching, rebuking, correcting and training in righteousness so that the servant of God may be thoroughly equipped for every good work." (2 Tim 3: 16-17)

Why then do we gloss over Scriptures on healing? I believe it is because we have not heard what the Word of God says about healing. We have not been taught these Scriptures. We have not heard sermons on these Scriptures. It's time to change that. The Greek word used in the New Testament for "repent" embodies the idea of changing the way you think. Let us repent, or change the way we think, about our biblical view of healing.

"What do you think?"

Matthew 21:28

1. What were you taught regarding praying for healing?

2. If someone were to ask you, could you give a testimony of a healing that you or a loved one received? (This will help build faith for the listener.)

God's Thoughts on Healing Your Body:

Psalms 41:3
The LORD nurses them when they are sick and restores them to health.

Isaiah 53:5
But he was pierced for our transgressions, he was crushed for our iniquities; the punishment that brought us peace was on him, and by his wounds we are healed.

Matthew 8:2-3

2 A man with leprosy came and knelt before him and said, "Lord, if you are willing, you can make me clean."

3 Jesus reached out his hand and touched the man. "I am willing," he said. "Be clean!" Immediately he was cleansed of his leprosy.

Matthew 9:20-22

20 Just then a woman who had been subject to bleeding for twelve years came up behind him and touched the edge of his cloak.

21 She said to herself, "If I only touch his cloak, I will be healed."

22 Jesus turned and saw her. "Take heart, daughter," he said, "your faith has healed you." And the woman was healed at that moment.

Matthew 12:15
Aware of this, Jesus withdrew from that place. A large crowd followed him, and he healed all who were ill.

Matthew 14:13-14
13 When Jesus heard what had happened, he withdrew by boat privately to a solitary place. Hearing of this, the crowds followed him on foot from the towns.

14 When Jesus landed and saw a large crowd, he had compassion on them and healed their sick.

Matthew 14:34-36
34 When they had crossed over, they landed at Gennesaret.

35 And when the men of that place recognized Jesus, they sent word to all the surrounding country. People brought all their sick to him

36 and begged him to let the sick just touch the edge of his cloak, and all who touched it were healed.

Matthew 15:29-31
29 Jesus left there and went along the Sea of Galilee. Then he went up on a mountainside and sat down.

30 Great crowds came to him, bringing the lame, the blind, the crippled, the mute and many others, and laid them at his feet; and he healed them.

31 The people were amazed when they saw the mute speaking, the crippled made well, the lame walking and the blind seeing. And they praised the God of Israel.

Luke 6:17-19
17 He went down with them and stood on a level place. A large crowd of his disciples was there and a great number of people from all

over Judea, from Jerusalem, and from the coastal region around Tyre and Sidon,

18 who had come to hear him and to be healed of their diseases. Those troubled by impure spirits were cured,

19 and the people all tried to touch him, because power was coming from him and healing them all.

Luke 13:11-13
11 and a woman was there who had been crippled by a spirit for eighteen years. She was bent over and could not straighten up at all.

12 When Jesus saw her, he called her forward and said to her, "Woman, you are set free from your infirmity."

13 Then he put his hands on her, and immediately she straightened up and praised God.

Scriptures Concerning Authority to Pray for Healing

Matthew 10:1

Jesus called his twelve disciples to him and gave them authority to drive out impure spirits and to heal every disease and sickness.

Mark 16:17-19

17 And these signs will accompany those who believe: In my name they will drive out demons; they will speak in new tongues;

18 they will pick up snakes with their hands; and when they drink deadly poison, it will not hurt them at all; they will place their hands on sick people, and they will get well."

19 After the Lord Jesus had spoken to them, he was taken up into heaven and he sat at the right hand of God.

John 10:10

The thief comes only to steal and kill and destroy; I have come that they may have life, and have it to the full.

Acts 10:38

how God anointed Jesus of Nazareth with the Holy Spirit and power, and how he went around doing good and healing all who were under the power of the devil, because God was with him.

Hebrews 13:8

Jesus Christ is the same yesterday and today and forever.

1 John 3:8

The one who does what is sinful is of the devil, because the devil has been sinning from the beginning. The reason the Son of God appeared was to destroy the devil's work.

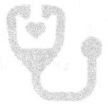

CHAPTER 12

A Word for A Patient

"I will instruct you and teach you in
the way you should go; I will counsel
you with my loving eye on you."
Psalms 32:8

As I was juggling between calls from patients, I heard our technician say, "Well, sir, you will have to go to talk to the Pharmacist at the Consult window." Generally, this situation takes precedence over most other matters and usually comes at a time of great hecticness.

I took a few lateral steps and popped into the private half-wall booth that separates me from the patient. A haggard looking man with droopy eyes looked intently at me with a hopeless despair. As he leaned both elbows on the small countertop of the consultation booth, he rubbed his face with the palms of his hands. "I can't sleep. Whatya got that can help?" God is good. He knew just what I needed to pull me away from the hectic pace and slow me down. This was another Divine Appointment arranged by the Great Physician.

My standard reply to such patient questions is "tell me more." This gives me a chance to corral all my loose mental marbles and to open my "inner ears" to the Holy Spirit. At this point, I usually pause long enough to ask Holy Spirit what He wants me to do. The patient said, "Almost every night I wake up around 11:30 p.m. or so, and I just lay there in bed and toss and turn. I might drift back off to sleep around 2 a.m. and am awake before 5. I can't go on like this. I need some rest. You have anything over the counter?"

With me, Holy Spirit is blunt. I receive short commands. Holy Spirit said to me, "Go talk with him." Immediately, I gave directions to the staff to hold my calls and that I will be back in a few minutes. The patient came over and we sat together at our soda fountain.

This is where the rubber meets the road. You either trust God and obey, or not. I started the conversation by saying these words that spilled out of my mouth without much thought. "I believe God is trying to get your attention. Do you spend time in prayer each day?" The patient's demeanor totally changed. He leaned back with an inquisitive look and raised eyebrows. "Well… I was really active in my prayer group at church, and then COVID hit. Then we stopped meeting."

The follow-up was easy. "Did you sleep well during that time?"

"Come to think of it, I did," he said as he nervously tumbled his thumbs over each other. I smiled, "Before we throw pills at the problem, I would encourage you to do this: when you wake up tonight at 11:30, get up and go sit in your chair and say, 'OK, God, what do you want to talk about?' I bet He has things He wants to discuss with you."

"That's a deal," the patient said.

I asked him if I could pray for him. He said yes and cradled his right hand in both of mine. "Thank You, God, that You care enough about us that You want to spend time with us. Please bless my new friend as he seeks You tonight." This counseling session was rung up as a No Sale. We stood and shook hands, and he left with a smile and a new purpose in his step.

A few weeks later, I was knee-deep in a patient's profile and happened to glance up to see my new friend. The look that people have after God touches them is unmistakable. His baggy eyes were almost normal again. His shoulders were square. His smile, victorious. He didn't say anything but just kept smiling at me. "Hi, Friend!" I called and left the pharmacy to go to the merchandise section where he was. We exchanged smiles and handshakes. "How are you doing?" I asked.

"You were right," came the reply, "God did have a lot to say!" I didn't ask what was said or any details. But he gave me a gift. "Thank you for taking time to talk to me. That's rare these days. I am resting just fine now."

"All glory to God!" is my standard response. He left the store smiling. And I was smiling as I went back to the pharmacy area. I sensed the affirmation of the Holy Spirit. God is so good. I glanced at the box of antihistamines on the shelf that I usually recommend for patients suffering from sleeplessness. "Maybe next time."

Analysis of this encounter reveals a stepwise progression. A patient had a need. I took time to go speak to him instead of just shouting out a remedy over the glass partition. I took time to listen to Holy Spirit. That's all the Holy Spirit needed. That guy could have walked into any pharmacy in town. I had never seen him before, nor have I seen him since. God sent him my way. That is humbling.

I encourage you to be obedient and sensitive to Holy Spirit as He directs people your way. Please understand that these patients likely drove past other suitable healthcare options to come see you. Holy Spirit directs them to you for a reason. That reason being that Holy Spirit knows you will be the hands and feet of Jesus to a hurting world.

"What do you think?"

Matthew 21:28

1. Describe an encounter that you have had with a patient which ended up with no medical treatment administered.

2. What is the primary takeaway for you in the above story?

Go Deeper

Hebrews 13:1-2
John 13:34-35
Philippians 2:3-4
Matthew 11:28-30
Psalm 32:8

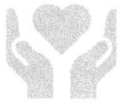

CHAPTER 13

NNP - Number Needed to Pray

"Do not quench the Spirit. Do not treat prophecies with contempt but test them all; hold on to what is good, reject every kind of evil.

1 Thessalonians 5:19-22

The Number Needed to Treat (NNT) value is a derived statistical measurement used to help determine the efficacy of a medication. Simply stated, the NNT relates how many patients must be treated with the medication for only one patient to get better who would not have gotten better without the medication. For example, an NNT of a cholesterol medication may be 15. If the "measurement" is fatal heart attack, then 15 patients must receive the medication to prevent one less fatal heart attack.

Even a brief glance at these numbers tells us that many more patients who take the medication will still experience the fatal heart attack. Only one person will live longer as a result, on average. The reality is that people take medications everyday on schedule and still die. However, folks continue to make doctor appointments and travel to big cities to see specialists. They stand in long lines waiting for their routine medications to be prepared. Adult children of elderly patients go to great lengths to ensure medical services, payment of bills, and delivery of medications are seamless. Very few patients decide to quit doctors and medications altogether when these might have no effect, or if news arrives of a loved one's passing.

Considering this devotion to doctors' offices and pharmacies, why are patients not as diligent in prayer? Why are we so apt to quit prayer when no immediate result is observed? Prayer is zero cost. Prayer does not need to be organized into daily containers. Prayer does not have deductibles to reach and expensive copays. Patients do not need to drive to big cities for prayer. Nevertheless, we all have the tendency to walk away from prayer when what we expect or hope for does not occur.

What would be the NNT for prayer? How many patients would you need to pray for to get better who would not be better without the prayer? This question leads us to consider what "get better" means. If we consider "get better" to mean "benefit", how many people would benefit from prayer? Would you agree that everyone would benefit in some way from prayer?

How often we hear, "Please pray for me." Is this simply a common benediction pronounced just before parting ways at the end of a conversation, or is it a plea from the heart? How many times have we said in response to that plea, "I will!" and then never do?

A primary human need is to be heard and understood. We want to know in our core that we are not alone, we are not aberrant, or the solitary example of some unusual person in the world. Prayer joins our hearts together seeking good. Prayer unites us in seeking the heart of the Father and the goodness of the Father.

I have seen in my practice the impact of one-on-one prayer. Almost everyone who received prayer from me or my staff left "better." Tears are an obvious sign that the Holy Spirit has touched someone whether or not they are a believer in King Jesus. Hugs and smiles are closely correlated to "getting better" as well. When a person's spirit is uplifted, they know they are not alone and that someone cares for them.

Compassion is the key here. No longer are they Chart Number R134529 or the 3:45 p.m. appointment, but they are a soul yearning for wholeness and peace and for the chance to chase their dreams and see their grandchildren grow. I believe the NNT for prayer — the NNP — approaches 1. Each person who receives prayer leaves with more hope, faith, and love than before the prayer. And you as the practitioner are bolstered and strengthened to continue pouring out love and attention to other patients.

Some well publicized evangelists have damaged the privilege of praying for the sick. We have witnessed long sermons whipped up by emotion and evangelists snatching folks out of wheelchairs and watching the newly healed sprint across the stage. This type of theatrics leaves us with a metallic taste in our mouths, and so we do not pray. While genuine healings do occur in the above scenarios, this method is not the only one which will produce "effectual fervent prayer [that] availeth much."

I call forth the plans of the Lord in your medical practice to pray for your patients. Allow Holy Spirit, who knows God's secret thoughts, to guide your prayers. Short prayers are perfectly fine. Calmly spoken prayers are perfectly fine. Most of my prayer times with patients are under one minute. But the results are long lasting. Would you invest one minute of your time for the well-being of your patient?

Do your own NNP (Number Needed to Pray) analysis. Prayer changes things. Prayer reduces depression and lifts spirits because of the promise of Isaiah 55:11, "... so is my word that goes out from my mouth: It will not return to me empty but will accomplish what I desire and achieve the purpose for which I sent it." Keep a diary of your prayers and refer to it when patients return to your practice. Watch and see what the Father will do through your willingness to pray for your patients.

"What do you think?"

Matthew 21:28

1. What are your thoughts on the statistical measurement of the Number Needed to Treat and developing your own Number Needed to Pray measurement?

2. How has this chapter helped you realize the effectiveness of prayer and the importance of prayer?

Go Deeper

1 Corinthians 2:11

Matthew 4:23

Luke 9:6

Psalm 145:8-9

John 14:15

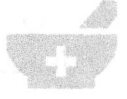

CHAPTER 14

Meet The Patient Where Their Faith Is

"Again, truly I tell you that if two
of you on earth agree about anything
they ask for, it will be done for
them by my Father in heaven."

Matthew 18:19

"Now faith brings our hopes into reality and becomes the foundation needed to acquire the things we long for. It is all the evidence required to prove what is unseen." (Heb. 11:1 TPT). The traditional King James Version puts it this way: "Now faith is the substance of things hoped for, the evidence of things not seen."

This chapter aims to present another key ingredient of faith: evidence.

As with the Number Needed to Treat idea presented earlier, this chapter is designed to help our "Evidence Based Medicine" colleagues see the proof and tangible aspects that faith embodies. Faith is an entity that can be grasped by the heart. It is the notion that what we have faith for is something that we know to be true and factual. It is presently, however, out of our field of vision and touch. It is the conviction that we will possess that entity one day.

I remember the doctor's appointment in which my wife's pregnancy was confirmed. It was evidence of a new life being created and knitted together in her womb. We could not see or touch our baby, but we beamed with smiles and warmth knowing it was only a matter of time dictated by natural processes set in motion by the Father.

Evidence also knits together the ideas and expectations of our patient's prayer outcomes. When our patients ask us to pray for them, there is a mental picture that the patient has of what the outcome of the answered prayer will look like. Our responsibility is to nurture that evidence, that faith, with our patient to achieve what they desire from prayer.

I have learned to pray at the level where a patient's faith is at the time when the patient asks for a specific desired outcome through prayer. I come into agreement with the patient as to what they want. I meet the patient where his or her faith is. If the patient has expressed what they want, it is risky to overpower them with some prayer that does not align with their level of faith or belief. The faith of the patient is increased when the specific prayer generated from the patient is answered rather than a prayer I have talked them into praying.

One of our patients suffered a huge gash on his left leg as a result of a fall from standing on the back of a golf cart. After attention and care from the Urgent Care doctor, this wound was treated with antibiotic ointment and wrapped with non-stick gauze. This patient is as devout a Christian as I know. If it's in the Bible, he knows the passage and can tell you where to find it.

When he asked for prayer for his deep wound in his leg, I was expecting him to ask for complete healing. Instead, he wanted me to pray that the follow-up visit to the doctor would go well and for the leg to continue to heal. I agreed to do so.

I did not think that He was asking God to do something that would not ordinarily happen. But I kept my mouth shut and smiled in agreement. I came into agreement with him as requested. His leg continued to heal rapidly and finally completely. His faith was strengthened.

Jesus mentioned several times in the Scriptures that the faith of the patient made them well. A well-known story is that in Luke 8:48, "And he said to her, Daughter, your faith has made you well." (ESV). Another example is in Luke 17:19, when Jesus healed 10 lepers and only one returned to give Him thanks, Jesus said, "Rise and go; your faith has made you well."

We need to meet our patients at their faith level, not ours. We may want to pray for the miracle healing or the regrowth of an organ, but if our patient's faith is not there, we will run them over and cause more damage than benefit. The key point is to come into agreement with the patient about the desired outcome. What we desire or think is possible is irrelevant, and perhaps counterproductive. As Matthew 18:19 states, "Again, truly I tell you that if two of you on earth agree about anything they ask for, it will be done for them by my Father in heaven."

I have foolishly bucked this scripture and decided to pray something other than what the patient requested. Only frustration and lack of results were the outcomes. Come into agreement with your patient. If their prayers are answered in the manner they pray, this will increase their faith, yield a closer walk with Jesus, and lead to testimony and witnessing of God's goodness.

Be careful not to impose your own agenda into the prayer, but rather come into agreement with the patient. This agreement also forms a bond between the two of you that means a great deal to the patient. After all, the patient is asking you for prayer.

You are to be as Jesus was to the blind man – a servant. In Mark 10:51, Jesus asks, "What do you want me to do for you?" This is the request of a servant, not the request of someone with an unmovable agenda. Meet your patient at their faith level. Perhaps you may even learn something and see God move in a way you never have before.

"What do you think?"

Matthew 21:28

1. Is there a point in this chapter on which you disagree? What is it, and why?

2. How would you approach a patient who wishes for God to answer a prayer that is not what you would have prayed for in that circumstance?

Go Deeper

Amos 3:3
1 Corinthians 1:10
Philippians 4:6
Romans 14:19
1 Peter 3:8

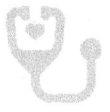

Chapter 15

Idiopathic Disease

"And a woman was there who had
been subject to bleeding for twelve
years. She had suffered a great deal
under the care of many doctors and
had spent all she had, yet instead of
getting better she grew worse."

Mark 5: 25-26

The Merriam Webster Dictionary defines the
term idiopathic as, "arising spontaneously or
from an obscure or unknown cause." We have
all encountered patients who seem bewil-
dered with the sudden emergence of an illness.

Generally, all signs and symptoms are normal. But for some reason, the patient is suffering. These diseases are from unknown origins for seemingly unknown reasons.

These diseases arise spontaneously. Out of nowhere. At this point, what do practitioners normally do? The answer is to pursue the most likely cause. Many times, this approach is void of results. I am reminded of a patient who asked me for a recommendation for his persistent heartburn. He previously tried famotidine and ranitidine over the counter with no effect. Even the most common prescription medications did not help.

As it turns out, he was suffering from stress that presented as heartburn as a result of having an extramarital affair. In this instance, I doubt any medication would have helped. What he needed was confession and repentance. The cause of his disease was spiritual. Science would call it idiopathic. Disciples of Jesus would see the root cause and help liberate him.

As you see patients in your practice and come across a case that is eventually classified as idiopathic, it is a good chance this is a case of self-sabotage of some nature. A careful and prayerful approach should be taken if you intend to probe this area. In my experience, I have simply paused and asked the patient, "Is there anything that you would like prayer for?"

As always, follow the lead of the Spirit of God. "The Spirit blows where it wills, and who can tell where it is going?" (John 3:8). Always ask, "Holy Spirit, what do you want me to do in this instance?" Usually, the patient must ask forgiveness for a trespass or forgive those who trespassed against them. Sound familiar?

Often, we encounter the temptation to build dogma, liturgy, and a recipe in our prayers. For example, we pray and observe a wonderful miracle to a deserving patient. Then, we turn into baseball managers who are known for their superstitions and quirky routines. We begin to wear the same shoes and clothes, drive to work the same way, pray in the same cadence with the exact same words. We turn the move of God into a recipe. With a recipe, now we do not need God's interference with our program. We have the secret code which we can pronounce over the patient and expect to see amazing miracles, right?

"Take the staff, and you and your brother Aaron gather the assembly together. Speak to that rock before their eyes and it will pour out its water. You will bring water out of the rock for the community so they and their livestock can drink." (Num. 20:8). Here, we see a scenario identical to one that occurred almost 40 years earlier in Exodus 17:5-7. Moses has seen how this plays out and moves ahead with the striking-the-rock routine. Only this time, God had told Moses to take the staff but speak to the rock.

Although God caused water to pour out, He was not pleased with Moses. "But the LORD said to Moses and Aaron, 'Because you did not trust in me enough to honor me as holy in the sight of the Israelites, you will not bring this community into the land I give them.'" (Num. 20:12). Hebrews 10:31 says, "It is a dreadful thing to fall into the hands of the living God." As a result of not listening to Holy Spirit or seeking what He was doing in this instance,

Moses got it wrong. He lost his ticket to the promised land.

It is God's business and prerogative to operate and move as He wishes. Thus, it is imperative to find out what He is doing and get in on His plan, instead of relying on old wineskins from last time to hold the new wine of the present. When praying for your patients with idiopathic illnesses, there are times in which you will not have a specific target on which to aim your prayers. I would recommend a prayer of blessing and praying for your patient to know the love of the Father. In this instance, display the love of the Father to your patient and allow Holy Spirit to do the convicting if any is needed.

"What do you think?"

Matthew 21:28

1. Relate an experience regarding one of your patients with an idiopathic disease.

2. Other than more medical tests, how did you handle this scenario? What would you do differently considering the information in this chapter?

Go Deeper

Proverbs 28:13
Psalm 69:5
Psalm 139:23-24
Jeremiah 16:17
Luke 12:2

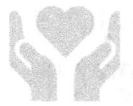

CHAPTER 16

Start Praying and Do Not Quit

"My sheep listen to my voice; I know them, and they follow me."

John 10:27

If you are a disciple of Jesus, you must realize that Jesus commanded us to pray for the sick. In the gospel of Matthew, Jesus uses the imperative tense. "Heal the sick, raise the dead, cleanse those with leprosy, drive out demons. Freely you have received; freely give." (Matt. 10:8). In the gospel of John, Jesus states it plainly, "If you love Me, keep my commands." (Jn. 14:15). This may raise our eyebrows in disbelief. What, me pray for someone? I can't pray over someone. That is not my personality.

It is important to note, Jesus only became angry with the church elite. One of the reasons was their lack of compassion. "Woe to you Pharisees, because you give God a tenth of your mint, rue and other kinds of garden herbs, but you neglect justice and the love of God." (Lk. 11:42). Allow compassion to grow in you for your patients. Put yourself in their position. Share their pain and try to understand their plight.

If you are new to the idea of praying for your patients, simply ask if you can pray for them. What the patient hears is that you are willing to help bear their burden of pain. You are willing to go to Father God and cry unto Him on their behalf. Every few people will turn you down and many will welcome prayer.

The next step does not involve a recipe. It is Holy Spirit led. You simply invite the Holy Spirit into the room and listen to Him as He gives you the words to say. Stop praying when

He stops giving you words. The length of prayer does not matter, but rather the sincerity.

The hardest ask is the first ask. Just start. Ask the patient if you can pray for them. You will see their countenance change and perhaps a tear. You are telling them, "You matter to me, and you matter to God. Let's talk to Father God about this."

As a Praying Practitioner, you represent Jesus to the patient in a manner that perhaps they have never seen. Nonjudgmentally. Compassionately. Empathetically. You carry within you the Grace of our Lord Jesus Christ. Who lights a candle and hides it under a bushel basket? This is a bad idea as the basket may catch on fire! You should instead let your good works be evident to your patient and thereby give glory to God. (Matt. 5:15-16). This cannot happen until you take the initiative and ask to pray for your patient.

That tug that you feel in your belly is the Holy Spirit wooing you to intercessory prayer for the patient. That look of helplessness is the patient wooing you to intercessory prayer for them. As in a popular 1980's movie, you must stick out your foot and take the chance (Indiana Jones - The Last Crusade). When you do, the Holy Spirit will give you the words.

The second part of starting is not quitting. Think of a time when your alma mater lost to their archrival. Do you remember the disappointment? You spent money on tickets, fuel, parking, snacks, and your return was watching your team lose 45–0. Perhaps you became angry at the coach or the referees. Perhaps you spewed out angry words to whomever would listen. A momentary vow of "I will never go back!" was made. You chose not to wear your school colors for a while in your protest and embarrassment.

Then, the next season rolls around. You have renewed optimism for no reason other than it is the beginning of a new season that is full of possibilities. The coach is the same and much of the team is the same; however, you buy the tickets, the fuel, and the snacks. You pull out your school colors and wear them again with a smile. You remember good times with good friends when you were a student, and you cheer for your team.

You did not quit. You persevered. Why? The reason is expectancy. You expect this season will be different than last. Your optimism leads to increased faith that your team will win this season.

Let's pretend you were invited to play at The Augusta National Golf Club. Let's further dream that you finished your round of 18 holes with a final score of 68 with 4 birdies. This would be 4 under par. Would you be ecstatic, or what? I apologize to the non-golf readers. To get the full impact of this analogy, please ask the golfer closest to you. This would mean that you only birdied 22% of the holes. For the investment bankers out there, would you be happy with 22% return on investment?

Most of us are willing to quit praying for one another if we do not see the equivalent of 18 birdies or have a 100% return on investment. We must persevere and be persistent in our prayers. Jesus taught on this issue. "Then Jesus told his disciples a parable to show them that they should always pray and not give up" (Lk. 18:1). Please see the Go Deeper section of this chapter for the full reference. The nugget of truth is this: prayer is work and will require effort.

A prime reason we stop praying for others is that we are disappointed God did not answer the prayer just like we wanted. I remember a group of us gathered to fast for a precious young girl who was facing either a liver transplant or the end of life. We fasted for 3 days – nothing but water. On the third day, which was a Sunday, we gathered around this young girl, anointed her with oil, and prayed down the heavens for supernatural healing.

In just a few days, we heard that an exceptional match had been found for her liver! Our group was celebrating the goodness of God. Except for me. I was disappointed. I pulled one of my friends aside and expressed that I wanted complete healing – a brand new liver from the storehouses of God. My friend chastised me and said God will answer how He wants. We must celebrate His answer because He is always good.

I admit that this speech did not help. I mean, this is God we are talking about. He created by speaking a word. "Let there be..." Jesus commanded us to heal the sick (Matt. 10:8). James, who was Jesus' brother, said to anoint the sick and they would be healed. Apparently, my definition of "healing" was different than the rest of the group. This hindered my intercessory prayer life for a while. What was I missing? Like the disciples, I wanted to pull Jesus to the side and ask Him, "What went wrong here?"

As I reflect on this event many years ago, I presented a different prayer to God than the rest of the group. Unfortunately, I was not in agreement with them. The great news is the girl received the liver and is now an adult who is thriving. God is good all the time! However, He is God and I am not. His ways are higher than my ways and His thoughts higher than mine. This event taught me to pray unashamedly to the Father who is able to do exceedingly and abundantly more than I could even imagine – then leave the results to Him.

The point is, do not allow what you see as failures or delays in intercessory prayer to stymie your prayer life. Your task is to pray. After that, the results are not up to you. Father God has a million different ways to accomplish the answer to the prayer that we lift up to Him. We are not to make demands or tell God to answer in a certain way. His word will accomplish everything He wants, in the manner that He wants it. (Isa. 55:11).

"What do you think?"

Matthew 21:28

1. What was your first miraculous answer from Father God that one of your patients received? How did this affect your prayer life?

2. What is one obstacle to starting a habit of praying for your patients in your area of practice?

Go Deeper

Luke 18:1-5
1 Timothy 2:1
Ephesians 6:18
Micah 7:7
1 Thessalonians 5:16-18

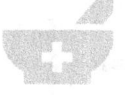

CHAPTER 17

How Do I Pray?

"One day Jesus was praying in a
certain place. When he finished,
one of his disciples said to him,
'Lord, teach us to pray, just as
John taught his disciples.'"

Luke 11:1

Hopefully by now, you are convinced and enthusiastic about praying for your patients. But you may not be accustomed to this and may not know where to start. Perhaps you are concerned about it getting weird or awkward. All you need is a blueprint on how to take the first step. A general outline is provided below, but the primary thing you need is to witness the first answer to a prayer that you prayed over a patient. Then, you will be unstoppable. I ask our Father who is in Heaven right now to answer your prayers in an amazing, supernatural way!

The first step is to start from a place of compassion. Artificial, plastic tree prayers will instantaneously be identified by the patient as contrived and fake. All the miracles of Jesus started from a place of compassion. Allow the fruit of the Spirit to help your heart become more compassionate. This fruit comes from The Vine who gives life. "I am the true vine, and my Father is the Gardener. He cuts off every branch in me that bears no fruit, while every branch that does bear fruit, He prunes so that it will be even more fruitful." (Jn. 15:1-2).

Ask the patient sincerely, "Do you mind if I pray for you?" Almost everyone, after they get over the shock of the question, says, "Sure." The next step is almost involuntary as we reach with our hands towards the patient. Ideally, we would like to place hands on the area that hurts. However, ask the patient if you may touch them. Do not assume that they would not mind. If the patient is of the opposite sex, be cautious. Either touch them on the top of the shoulder or ask their spouse, if present, to place their hand on the area of need, and then you place your hand on top of the spouse's hand. Do not give the devil a foothold by being careless in this arena. (Eph. 4:27).

It is now time to pray! Be led by the Holy Spirit who knows exactly what we should pray Rom. 8:26). In general, pray brief prayers and not a prayer that would qualify for the rebuke that Jesus mentioned in the Sermon on the Mount: "And when you pray, do not use vain repetitions as the heathen do. For they think that they will be heard for their many words." (Matt 6:7 NKJV). Develop your own style of prayer in terms of how you will start and end.

My wife prays God's Scriptures back to Him. For example, "Father, Your word says that where two or more are gathered, you are there. Father, Your word commands us to heal the sick. Father, You said whatever we ask in Your name, it will be done for us, so I ask…" This is an awesome method. Most of the time, I find myself in a conversation with Father God as I just summarize and speak out what the patient and I have been talking about. My scriptural basis is, "Truly I tell you, if anyone says to this mountain, 'Go, throw yourself into the sea' and does not doubt in their heart but believes that what they say will happen, it will be done for them." (Mk. 11:23, emphasis added).

Some friends of ours, when they pray, get straight to the point. "I command this TMJ pain to stop right now in the mighty name of Jesus." The point is, along with compassion, you must convey commitment, authority, and sincerity in your prayer. I strongly encourage you to end your prayer with a blessing for the patient. A typical one of mine is, "Thank you Father for hearing our prayer. I bless my friend and pray Your goodness and peace on them as you work in their life."

When Jesus gave the commandment to heal the sick, He did not give us a step-by-step formula. Neither did the Apostle Paul or any other New Testament author give us detailed instructions about how to do so. I believe this is intentional. This must be Spirit-led. The approach and content will likely vary each time. This is why it is vital to discern what the Spirit is saying and act accordingly.

Many times, praying for a patient will not occur to me as I discuss symptoms and medications with a patient until suddenly, the Holy Spirit nudges me to move into that area. Sometimes, I resist and His nudge becomes a heart pine 2x4 whacked over my head. The great news here is, the Spirit just wants to be invited in, and He will take care of the rest. When I get these strong nudges, I know the patient will be touched by God and will leave our practice site changed for the better.

How did Peter pray for the Lame Beggar just inside the Eastern Gate of the Temple Mount? He was brief and to the point. "Then Peter said, 'Silver or gold I do not have, but what I do have I give you. In the name of Jesus Christ of Nazareth, walk." (Acts 3:6). He was very economical with his words. He commanded that the man get up and walk. Just as Jesus did.

At the Pool of Bethesda, when Jesus healed the invalid, He said, "Get up! Pick up your mat and walk." (Jn. 5:8). Peter simply imitated Jesus. Peter utilized the authority given to him by Jesus. This direct method was also utilized by Jesus when He was tempted by the devil in the wilderness. (Matt. 4:1-11). There was no debate or discussion. The simple reply from Jesus after each temptation was to say, "It is written…"

Many of us are reluctant to command a healing to occur. However, this is what Jesus did and what Peter did. In Acts, Paul repeated this direct method. "He listened to Paul as he was speaking. Paul looked directly at him, saw that he had faith to be healed and called out, 'Stand up on your feet!' At that, the man jumped up and began to walk." (Acts 14:9-10). No need to beat the rug too much. Peter and Paul chose to exercise the authority that Jesus has given every believer. If you are a Christian, you have that authority also.

"What do you think?"

Matthew 21:28

1. How is your confidence level as you commit to pray for your patients? What is the most alarming issue to you regarding praying for your patients?

2. Will you commit to prayIng for your patients? If so, how will you share this with   your colleagues?

Go Deeper

Joshua 1:9
Isaiah 41:10
Matthew 28:20
Psalm 23:1
Jeremiah 29:11

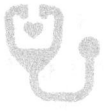

CHAPTER 18

Last Thoughts

"For God has not given us a
spirit of fear, but of power and
of love and of a sound mind."

2 Timothy 1:7

I pray that this book has helped you in many ways regarding the exciting opportunity to pray for the patients in your practice. Scripture and the will of Father God firmly support your decision to pray.

Our patients can take their meds and receive our prayers. Deuteronomy 29:29 states, "The secret things belong unto the Lord our God, but those things which are revealed belong unto us and to our children forever, that we may do all the words of this law." (KJV). Medical practice is a revealed thing! Medications are for us, not against us. Paul, from whom clothes that touched his skin healed patients (Acts 19), instructed Timothy to "stop drinking only water and use a little wine because of your stomach and frequent illnesses." (1 Tim. 5:23). Medications are a blessing from God.

So then, what about these secret things mentioned in the previous paragraph? Answers to prayers and the mysterious workings of the answers of prayers belong to God. We submit to God. We submit to His mercy, His judgements, and His authority. On occasion, prayers are not answered in the manner we want them answered. We have the prescription ready only for God's signature, but God is led by no man. He is sovereign. He decides. We praise Him and trust that He is always good.

Ask the Lord for a Divine Appointment each day at the office. Ask God to bring someone to you who needs a special touch from the Father. Ask God for heavenly insight, or words of knowledge (1 Cor. 12:8), about the situation, to guide your prayers and fully understand the present state of the one for whom you are praying.

I also encourage you to develop networks of practitioners who pray for their patients. Share stories of miracles with each other, as well as times when the answer was not what you asked. We all want to hear the testimonies of healings that will flow from your practice! "Let your light so shine before men, that they may see your good works, and glorify your Father which is in heaven." (Matt. 5:16 KJV).

May God richly bless your prayers!